MONKEYPOX:

The basic knowledge everyone should have about monkeypox.

By Pearl Miller

Table of Contents

Chapter 1: Introduction

In 2022, instances of monkeypox were recorded in several nations that are generally free of the disease. The majority of infections in this outbreak—but not all—are among males who engage in sexual activity with other men who have recently had intercourse with a new partner or partners. Fewer symptoms are frequently recorded than what was customarily observed in the past.

As of July 11, 2022, no connection has been made between the majority of cases that have been reported on an individual basis and travel from previously afflicted nations in Africa. In this epidemic, recent travel from different parts of the world is frequently mentioned.

We recognize that many people are worried about this epidemic, particularly those whose loved ones or communities have been impacted. The most crucial thing at this time is to educate those who are most susceptible to monkeypox and offer tips on how to stop future transmission between people. Additionally, public health professionals must be able to recognize, classify, and treat patients.

Because anybody can contract monkeypox and because stigmatization can weaken control efforts, no one must stigmatize anyone who is impacted by this outbreak. Consider providing instruments for monkeypox surveillance, readiness, and epidemic response in impacted nations.

To better understand how people are exposed to monkeypox, studies are being conducted in the afflicted nations. Medical attention is being given to people who are harmed, and public health initiatives are being established to stop the spread of the disease.

Chapter2: Describe monkeypox.

The monkeypox virus is the infection that causes monkeypox. It can transmit from animals to people since it is a viral zoonotic illness. It may also pass from one individual to another.

When a person comes into touch with an infected animal, they risk contracting monkeypox. Primates and rodents are examples of animal hosts. By staying away from unprotected contact with wild animals, especially those that are sick or dead, the chance of contracting monkeypox from them can be decreased (including their meat and blood). All items containing animal flesh or parts should be fully prepared before consumption in monkeypox-endemic nations.

The first case of human monkeypox in humans was discovered in 1970 in the Democratic Republic of the Congo in a 9-month-old boy in an area where smallpox had been eradicated in 1968. Since that time, the majority of human cases have been found in remote, rainforest parts of the Congo Basin, mainly in the Democratic Republic of the Congo, and cases have spread across central and west Africa.

Given that it affects the rest of the globe in addition to nations in west and central Africa, monkeypox is a disease of worldwide public health significance. The first monkeypox epidemic outside of Africa occurred in the United States of America in 2003, and contact with pet prairie dogs that had the disease was to blame. These pets had been kept with dormice and pouched rats from Ghana that were brought from the Gambia. Over 70 cases of monkeypox were brought on by this epidemic in the US.

Although no cases of humans spreading monkeypox to animals have been recorded, it is a possibility. Avoid close contact with all animals, including pets (such as cats, dogs, hamsters, gerbils, etc.), livestock, and wildlife, if you have proven or suspect monkeypox. Those who have monkeypox should take extra precautions while near non-human primates and rodents, which are known to be vulnerable to the monkeypox virus.

Chapter 3: monkeypox symptoms

Numerous symptoms and indicators are associated with monkeypox. While some people only have minor symptoms, others may experience more severe symptoms and require medical attention. Pregnant women, children, and anyone with impaired immune systems are at increased risk for serious illness or complications.

Monkeypox is most frequently characterized by fever, headache, muscular pains, back discomfort, lack of energy, and enlarged lymph nodes. A rash that can continue for two to three weeks develops as a result of or in conjunction with this. The face, palms of the hands, soles of the feet, eyes, mouth, throat, groin, and genital and/or anal parts of the body can all be affected by the rash. Lesions can number anywhere from one to thousands. Lesions start flat, fill with fluids, then crust over, dry up, and fall off, revealing a new layer of skin beneath.

Symptoms normally last two to three weeks and disappear on their own or with supportive treatment, such as fever-relieving drugs or painkillers. Until all lesions have crusted over, all scabs have fallen off, and a fresh layer of skin has developed below, a person is still contagious.

Anyone who may have monkeypox symptoms or who has come into touch with someone who has should contact or see a healthcare professional for guidance.

Chapter 4: Mode of transmission.

Close contact with someone who has a monkeypox rash, such as by face-to-face, skin-to-skin, mouth-to-mouth, or mouth-to-skin contact, including sexual contact, can transfer the disease from one person to another. Monkeypox sufferers are typically infectious until all of their lesions have crusted over, the scabs have gone off, and a new layer of skin has developed below. However, we are still discovering how long monkeypox sufferers are contagious.

Monkeypox virus contamination may occur in environments, such as when an infected individual touches items including clothing, bedding, towels, gadgets, and surfaces. If someone else comes in contact with these things, they might get sick. It's also possible to get a virus via clothing, bedding, or towels, or from breathing in skin flakes. Transmission of the fomite is what this is.

The virus can spread by direct contact with the mouth, respiratory droplets, and perhaps through short-range aerosols if there are ulcers, lesions, or sores in the mouth. Monkeypox transmission through the air may occur for unknown reasons, and research is being done to find out more.

The virus can also pass from a pregnant person to the fetus, from a newborn to a parent through intimate contact, or from a parent who has monkeypox to a kid.

Although cases of asymptomatic illness have been documented, it is unclear whether or not contagious diseases may be disseminated by asymptomatic individuals or by other body fluids. Semen has been confirmed to contain monkeypox viral DNA, however, it is unknown if semen, vaginal fluids, amniotic fluids, lactation, or blood may also transmit the illness. The question of whether persons may transmit monkeypox through the sharing of these fluids during and after symptomatic illness is now being researched.

Chapter 5: Is the monkey pox curable?

People who have monkeypox should heed their doctor's instructions. Treatment is typically not necessary because symptoms usually go away on their own. Analgesics and antipyretics, which are used to treat fever and discomfort, can be used to ease certain symptoms. Anyone suffering from monkeypox should drink enough fluids, eat healthfully, and get plenty of rest. Self-isolating individuals should take care of their mental health by engaging in activities that they find enjoyable and relaxing, staying in touch with loved ones via technology, engaging in physical activity if they feel well enough to do so while isolating, and seeking support for their mental health if necessary.

Monkeypox patients should refrain from scratching their rash and take care of it by washing their hands before and after handling the lesions and by keeping their skin dry and uncovered (unless they are unavoidably in a room with someone else, in which case they should cover it with clothing or a bandage until they can isolate again). Sterilized water or an antiseptic solution can be used to keep the rash clean. Mouth lesions can be treated with salt water rinses, while body lesions can be treated with warm Epsom salt and baking soda baths. Pain relief from oral and perianal lesions is possible with lidocaine application.

Products that may help treat monkeypox have been developed as a result of years of study on smallpox therapies. The European Medicines Agency authorized tecovirimat, an antiviral created to treat smallpox, in January 2022 to treat monkeypox. There is minimal experience using these medicines during a monkeypox outbreak. Because of this, gathering information to help with future usage is typically done in conjunction with their use.

Chapter 6: How to avoid getting monkeypox and how to protect others

By avoiding direct contact with people or animals that may be afflicted with the disease, you can lessen your chance of contracting monkeypox. Frequently clean and disinfect any areas that may have been infected with a virus from an infectious person. Keep yourself aware of the prevalence of monkeypox in your community and be upfront with anyone you come into close contact with (particularly during sexual activity) about any symptoms you or they may be experiencing.

By obtaining medical assistance and keeping to yourself until you have been examined and tested, you may take precautions to protect others if you believe you may have monkeypox. You should keep to yourself if you have monkeypox until all of your lesions have crusted over, the scabs have come off, and a new layer of skin has developed below if you have monkeypox that has been diagnosed as probable or proven. You won't be able to spread the infection to others as a result of this. Ask your health professional for guidance on whether you should isolate yourself at home or a medical institution. Use condoms as a precaution while having sexual contact for 12 weeks after you have recovered until more is known regarding the transfer of sexually transmitted diseases through sexual fluids.

If you have been in close contact with someone who has monkeypox or has been in a location where the virus may have been present, keep a watchful eye out for symptoms for 21 days following your last exposure. As much as possible, avoid having close personal interactions with others, but if it's necessary, let them know that you've just been exposed to monkeypox.

For guidance, evaluation, and medical attention, speak with your healthcare professional if you believe you may be experiencing monkeypox symptoms. If you can, keep yourself alone until you learn the results of your exam. Keep your hands clean.

If you test positive for monkeypox, your doctor will give you advice on how to treat the infection, whether you should isolate yourself at home or in a hospital.

Recently, a vaccination for monkeypox was licensed. For people who are at risk, several nations advise immunization. For the smallpox illness, which has been eliminated, better and safer vaccinations have been developed. These vaccines may also be helpful for monkeypox. One of these has been authorized for use in monkeypox prophylaxis. Only those who are vulnerable should be thought about getting vaccinated, such as those who have had intimate contact with someone who has monkeypox. At this time, mass immunization is not advised.

Although the smallpox vaccination is protective against monkeypox in the past, there is currently minimal information on the efficacy of more recent smallpox/monkeypox vaccines in preventing monkeypox in clinical settings and the field. It will be possible to quickly generate new data on the efficacy of these vaccinations in various contexts by examining the usage of monkeypox vaccines wherever they are used.

Currently, little is known about the duration of immunity following monkeypox infection. The extent to which having had monkeypox in the past confers protection against subsequent infections and for how long, if at all, are still unclear. Even if you've previously had monkeypox, you should take every precaution to prevent re-infection.

You can safeguard others by taking on the role of designated caregiver if you have had monkeypox in the past and someone in your home has it currently. This is because you are more likely than others to have some immunity. To prevent contracting an infection, you should still take all necessary precautions.

www.ingramcontent.com/pod-product-compliance
Lightning Source LLC
LaVergne TN
LVHW052117160826
845678LV00015B/3596

* 9 7 9 8 8 4 4 2 1 2 9 9 4 *